Aliyah M. Moore would like to thank the following people
for their generous and knowledgeable contributions:

Beth K. Thielen, MD, PhD
Division of Pediatric Infectious Diseases and Immunology
Department of Pediatrics
University of Minnesota Medical School

A&M A&K, S&C.

Edited by Danielle Amir-Lobel
Illustrated by Georgina Cahill

Illustrations credited to Yana Bondaruk:
Woman wearing a mask Page 1
Yogurt, cheese, and bread Page 7
Close-up of child coughing into her mask Page 17

THE WORLD KEEPS GOING AND TOGETHER WE WILLL TO:
A CHILDREN'S BOOK ABOUT THE CORONAVIRUS AND OTHER GERMS

Published by Aliyah M. Moore

Excerpted information on COVID-19 excerpted from the Centers for Disease Control and Prevention website, provided for informational purposes only.

Aliyah M. Moore, Author
THE WORLD KEEPS GOING AND TOGETHER WE WILL TO:
A CHILDREN'S BOOK ABOUT THE CORONAVIRUS AND OTHER GERMS
ALIYAH M. MOORE

ISBN: 978-0-578-80012-7

The World Keeps Going and Together We Will Too

A children's book about the coronavirus and other germs.

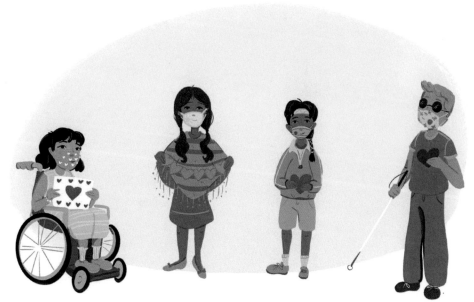

By Aliyah M. Moore

What's going on in the world today may be a little difficult to understand but always remember that, no matter where we come from and what we look like on the outside, our hearts are all the same. Right now, we may have to wear face masks to cover our faces, but that doesn't mean we have to cover our hearts. Let's work together to keep ourselves and others around us healthy.

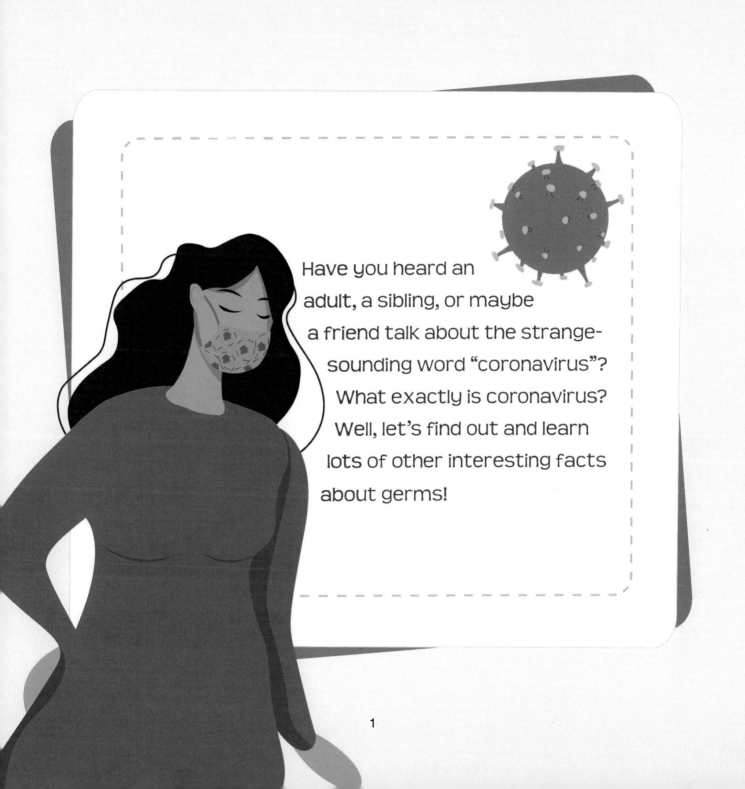

Have you heard an adult, a sibling, or maybe a friend talk about the strange-sounding word "coronavirus"? What exactly is coronavirus? Well, let's find out and learn lots of other interesting facts about germs!

1

Coronavirus is a virus that circulates among humans and animals, and there are seven different types of coronaviruses.

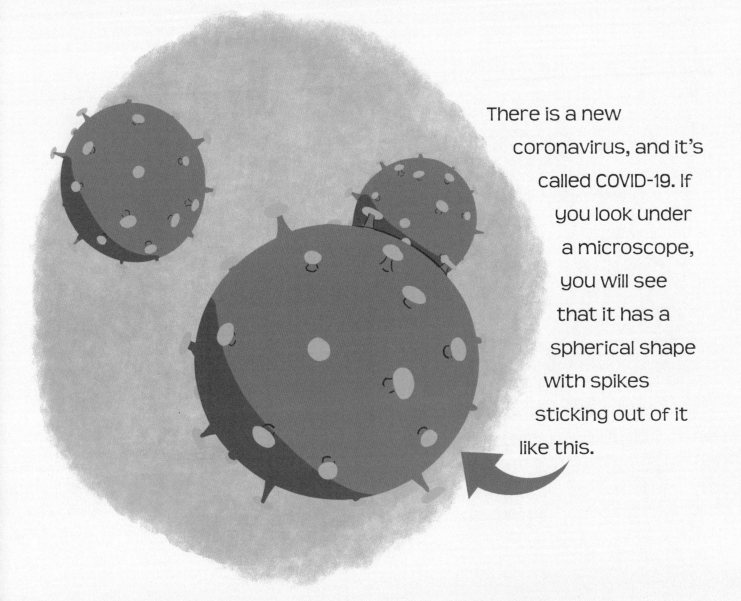

There is a new coronavirus, and it's called COVID-19. If you look under a microscope, you will see that it has a spherical shape with spikes sticking out of it like this.

This is
Sergeant Corona.
He is a
coronavirus.

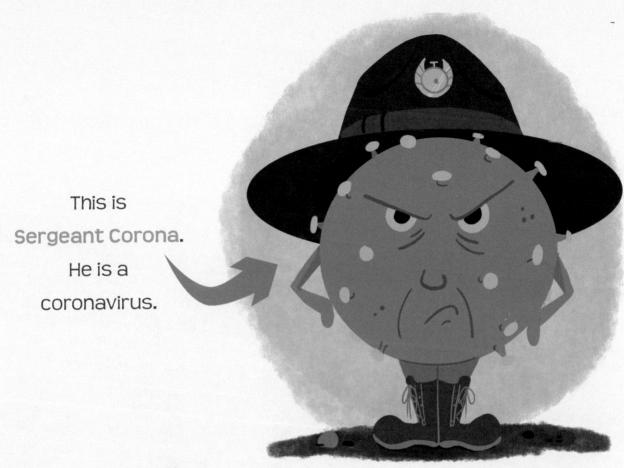

In Spanish, **'corona'** means
crown, and, as you can
see, Sergeant Corona looks
like a crown with spikes.

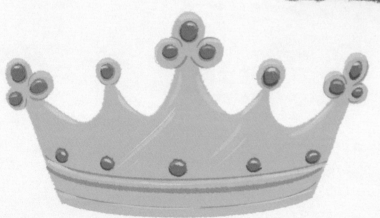

3

Meet Sergeant Corona's troops. Towards the end of 2019, Sergeant Corona gathered his troops together and formed a new group.

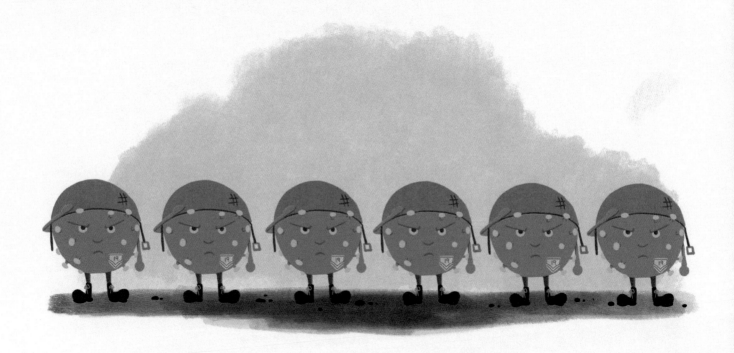

He named them "The COVIDs ."

Let's break it down.

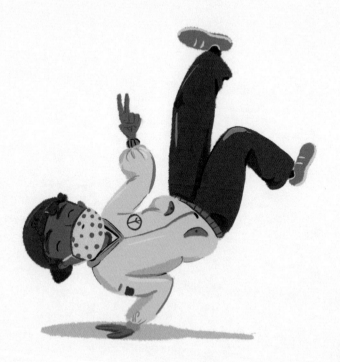

If you take the Spanish word 'corona' and add the word 'virus' to the end of it, what do you get? Coronavirus!

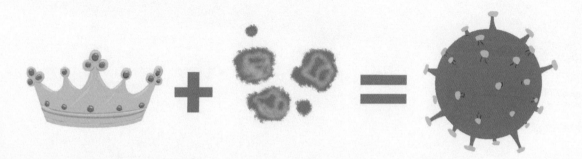

Viruses are a type of germ. There are many different kinds of germs in the world. Some germs are good and others are bad. Germs can be found just about anywhere-like on your body, on surfaces, in food, or in the air. But, you have to look through a microscope to see them because they are very tiny, so tiny that they are invisible to the eye.

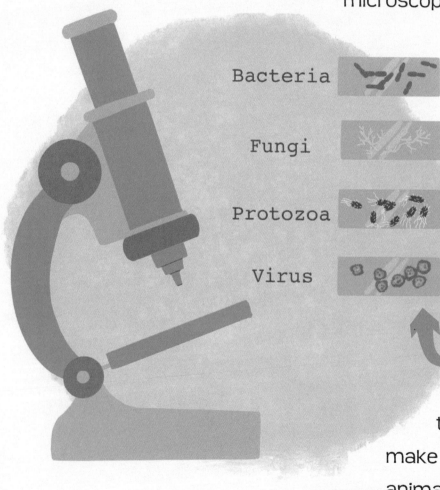

Bacteria

Fungi

Protozoa

Virus

These are the four major types of germs that can sometimes make people, plants, *and* animals sick.

6

Viruses and other bad germs can be gross because, once they are inside our bodies, they can make us feel sick. To stay healthy, you want to avoid the bad germs and instead try to look out for the good germs.

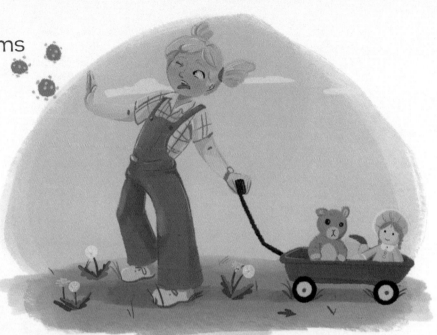

Certain foods like yogurt, cheese, and bread contain friendly bacteria, or germs, that can be good for your body. These germs can help improve the way food is digested in the body and provide many more positive boosts.

Sergeant Corona and his troops are some of these bad germs. In fact, Sergeant Corona has been up to no good! Everyday he sends out his troops to travel all around the world, and there are just too many of them to count!

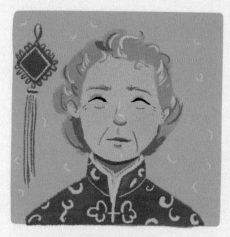 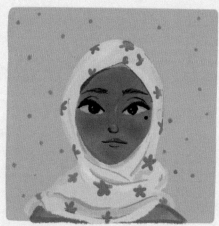 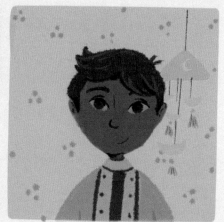

Their evil plan is to make people sick. In fact, they have already made a lot of people very sick. The COVIDs will make anyone sick no matter where you come from or what you look like.

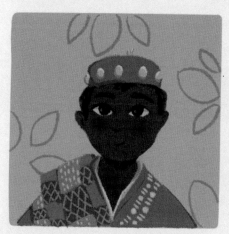 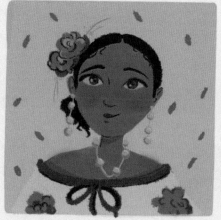 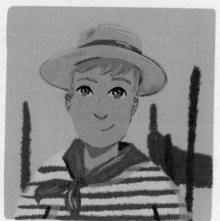

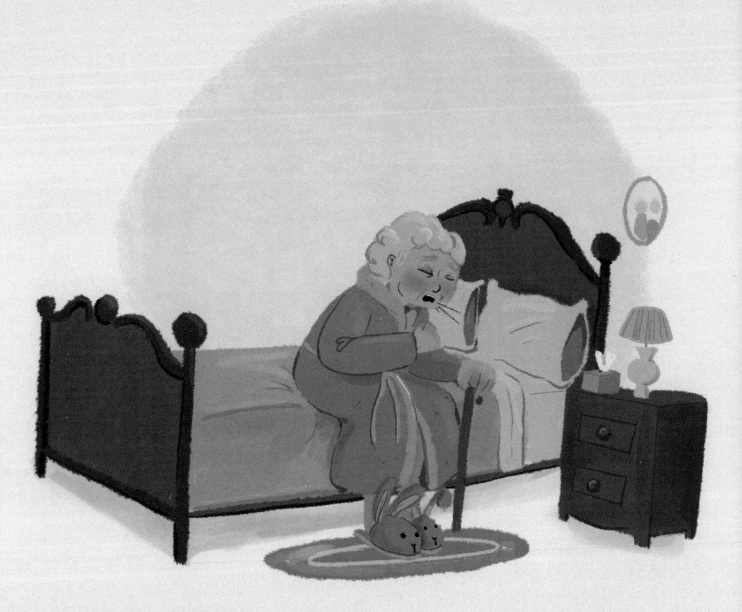

In particular, The COVIDs attack the most vulnerable people who already have medical conditions or are older adults.

How do The COVIDs and other germs spread? When someone who is sick coughs or sneezes, tiny droplets which contain germs fly out of their nose and mouth and into the air. Then they fly over onto the people and surfaces nearby. If those tiny droplets land on your eyes or mouth, or if you breathe them in, those germs enter your body. Once inside, their plan may be to make you feel sick next.

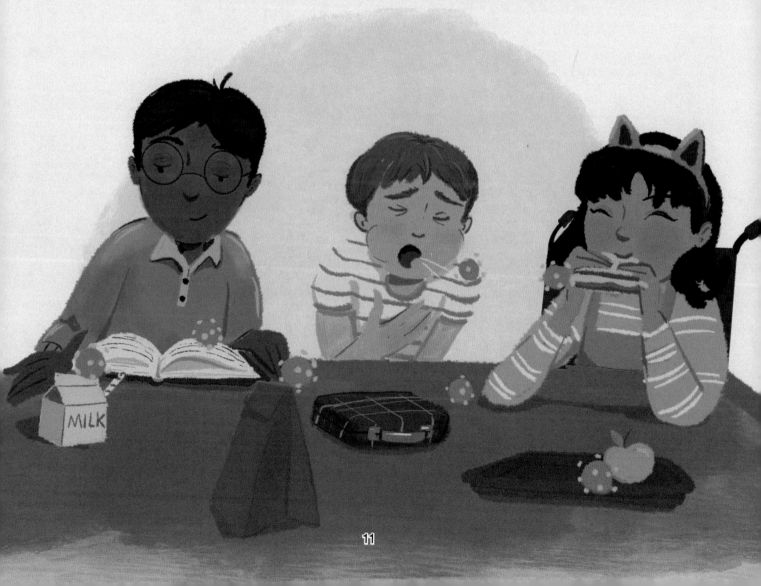

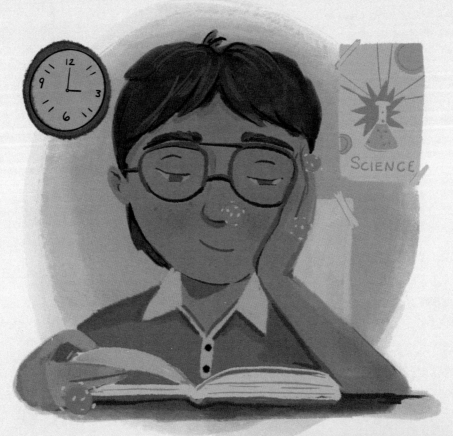

If we touch a surface that The COVIDs or germs are hiding on, they will crawl onto our hands and wait till we touch our eyes, ears, noses, or mouths, which they like to sneak into.

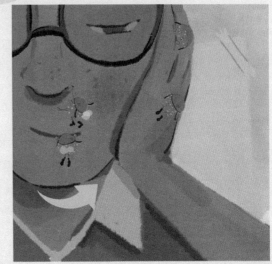

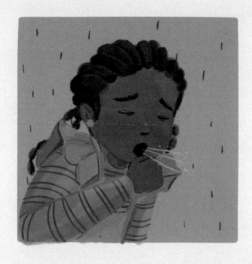

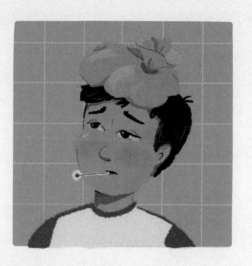

Different germs can make you feel different things. Once The COVIDs creep into our bodies, they can make us cough, ahem, ahem. Weeze. Feel very, very warm and really, really tired. But, in some cases, The COVIDs can hide inside of us without making us feel sick. Some people who have the new coronavirus, COVID-19, may feel no symptoms. However, they can still spread it to others, just like infected people who experience symptoms.

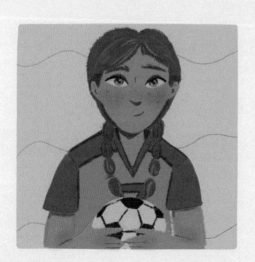

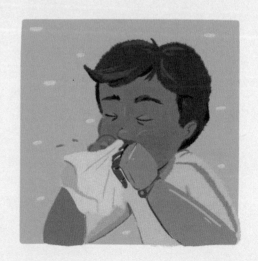

Doctors and scientists around the world are on a mission to stop Sergeant Corona and The Covids for good. They are working together to develop medicines and treatments to help people who become infected with The COVIDs get better more quickly. They have also successfully developed different types of COVID-19 vaccines! These vaccines will help prevent The COVIDs from getting people sick.

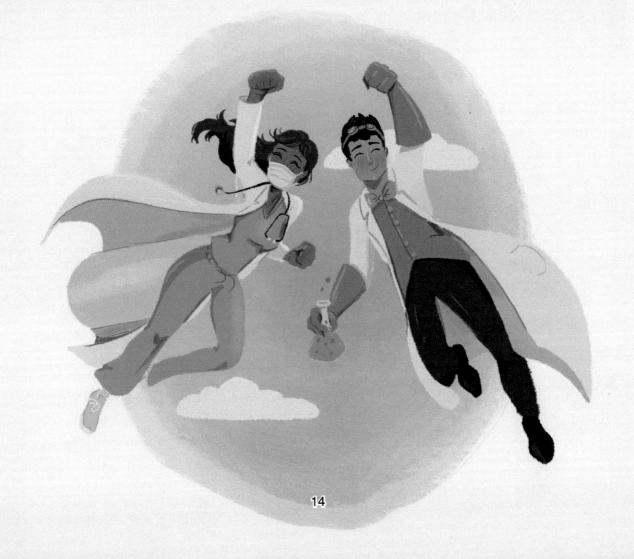

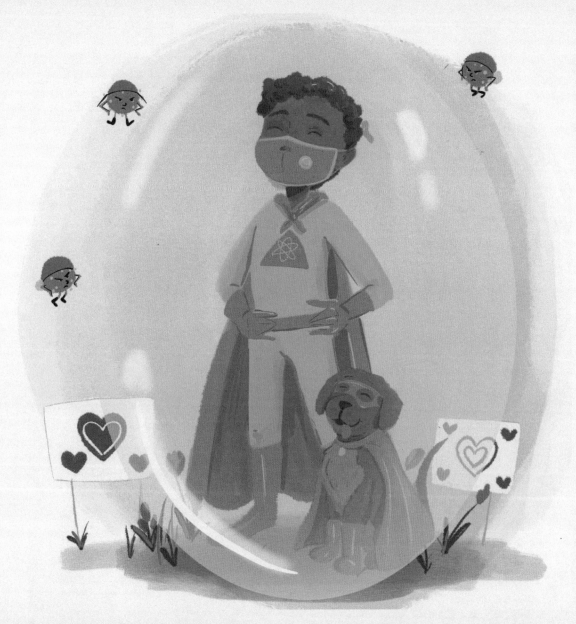

In the meantime, let's learn about some of the essential steps we can take to protect ourselves, our families, and our friends from getting sick from The COVIDs and any other icky germs out there!

Step 1:

Sneeze and cough into your elbow or a tissue, making sure to wash your hands after.

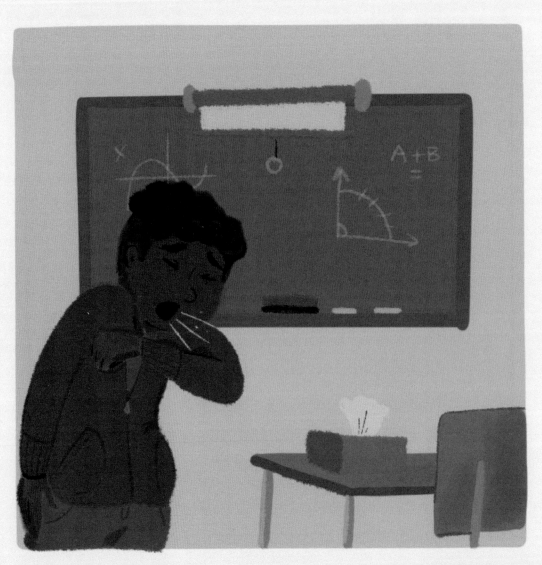

Step 2:

It's important to wear a face mask in public or around other people who don't live in your house. It may feel a little uncomfortable wearing them, but certain face masks could help protect you and others around you from getting sick.

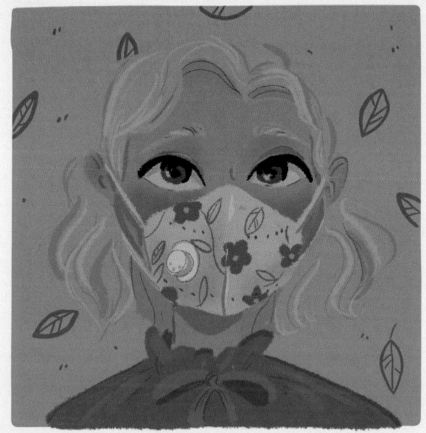

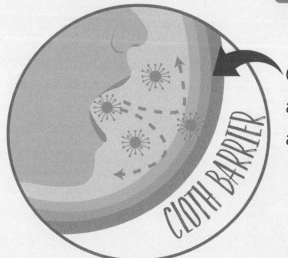

CLOTH BARRIER

Germs will have trouble sneaking in and out your nose and mouth if you are covering them up.

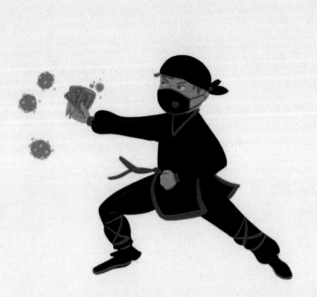

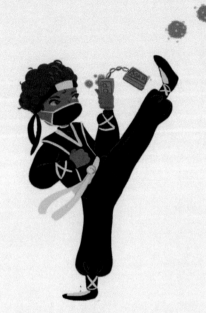

But face masks do more than just keep you safe—you can also make them fun by pretending you're a secret ninja fighting off icky germs!

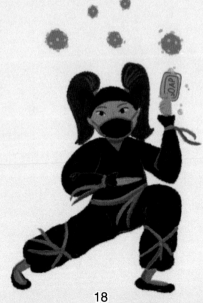

Step 3:

Wash your hands often for at least 20 seconds with soap and water. When should we wash our hands? We should always wash them carefully before and after touching our face, eating, using the bathroom, and playing outside.

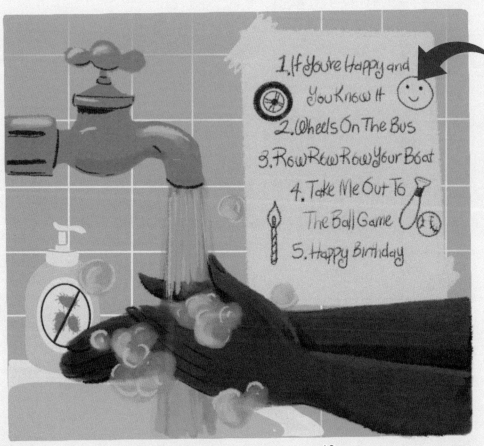

You can also sing your favorite song to pass the time!

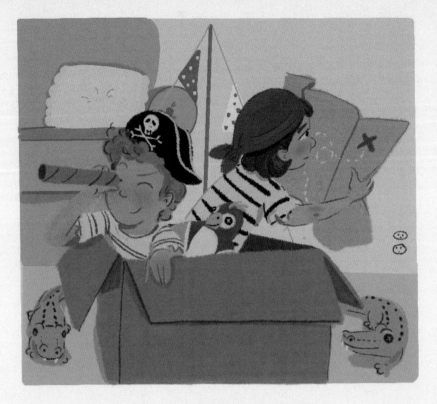

Step 4:

Stay at home and make it fun! Here's an idea for a fun activity to try at home:

- ☐ Find an old Halloween pirate costume or create one with whatever you have in your closet.
- ☐ Build a pirate ship out of a shipping box and pretend the floor is water.
- ☐ Grab a paper towel roll to use as a telescope.
- ☐ Set sail to sea in search of hidden treasures!

Arr! Good luck with your adventure matey.

Step 5:

Lastly, let's try to socially distance, or physically distance, ourselves from our friends and family members who don't live in our house, in order to keep everyone healthy.

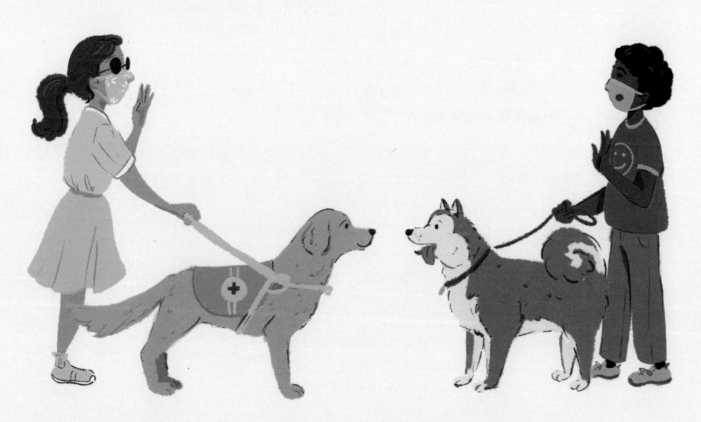

Physical distancing means maintaining a safe space of six feet apart or more from one another while still maintaining a social connection. A six-foot distance is like the length of a door, a cow, or two large dogs standing between you and the other person.

When physically distancing, let's all pretend we are in a bubble that surrounds us. This bubble is going to work as a shield to help protect you from The COVIDs and any other icky germs getting too close to you.

But you have to make sure to keep a safe space of six feet or more from one another so your bubble shields don't crash and go... POP!

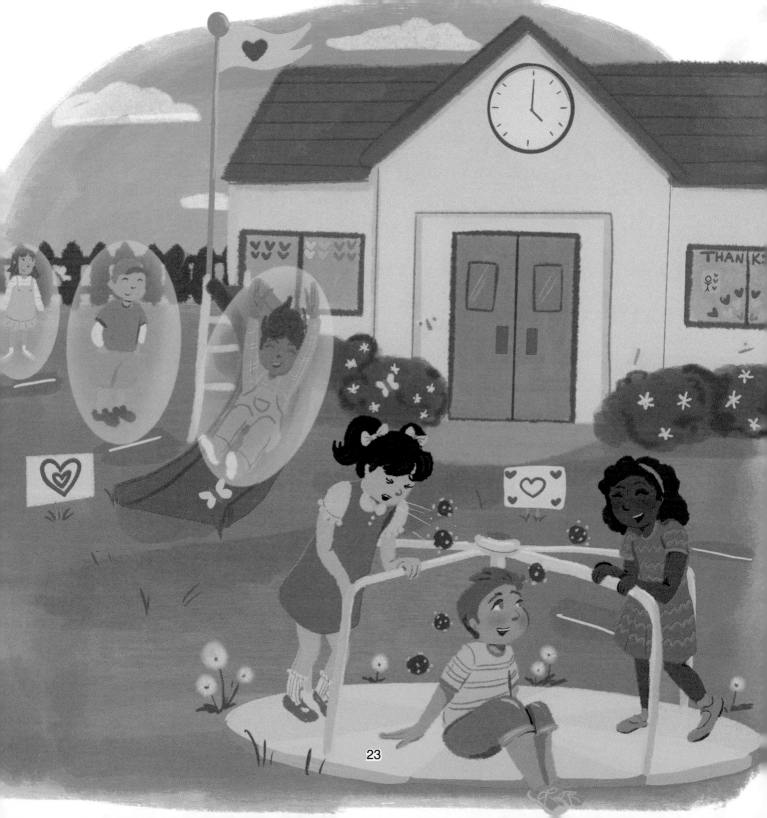

23

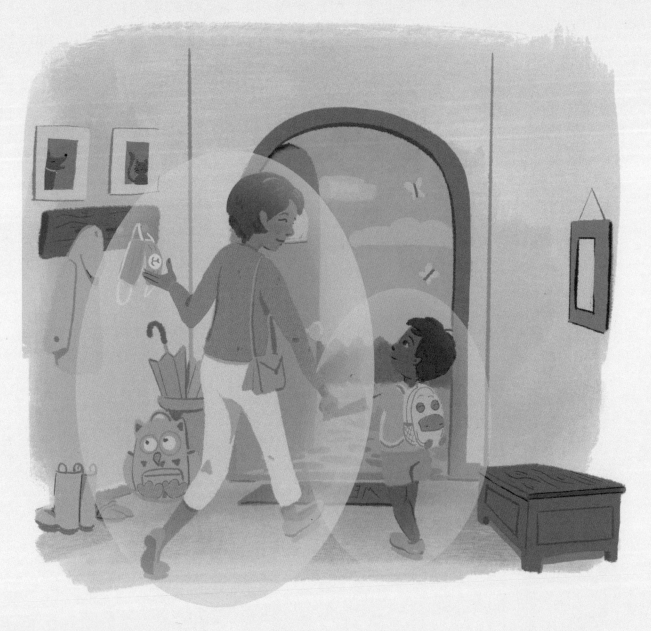

When you go to school or meet up with a group of friends, don't forget to wear your bubble shields.

If you practice these essential steps, you'll not only protect your own health but the health of everyone around you as well. Plus, your friends will see how cool you are for practicing these steps, and they will want to do the same! Cool means being yourself because being yourself never goes out of style.

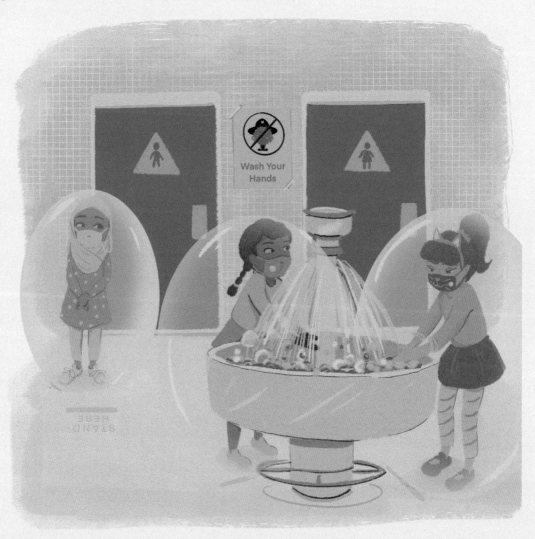

A lot of grown ups in your community and around the world are working hard to come up with new ways to protect you from getting sick. But what happens if you do get sick? Don't worry! Remember there are doctors and nurses who can help.

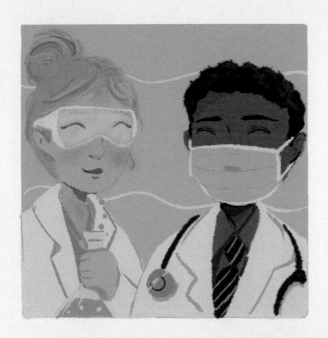

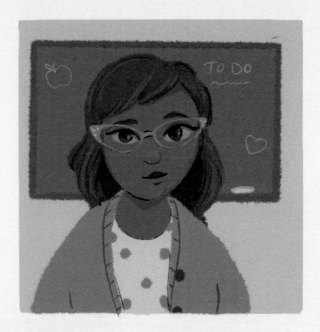

And that's worth smiling for!

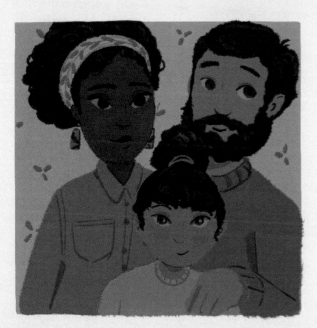

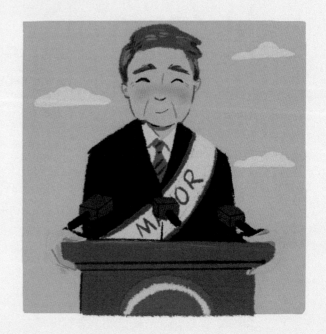

Friendly reminder: Be kind to one another.

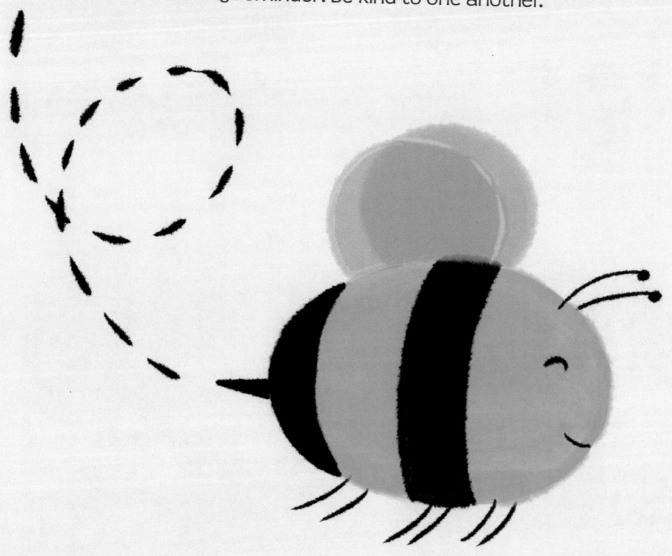

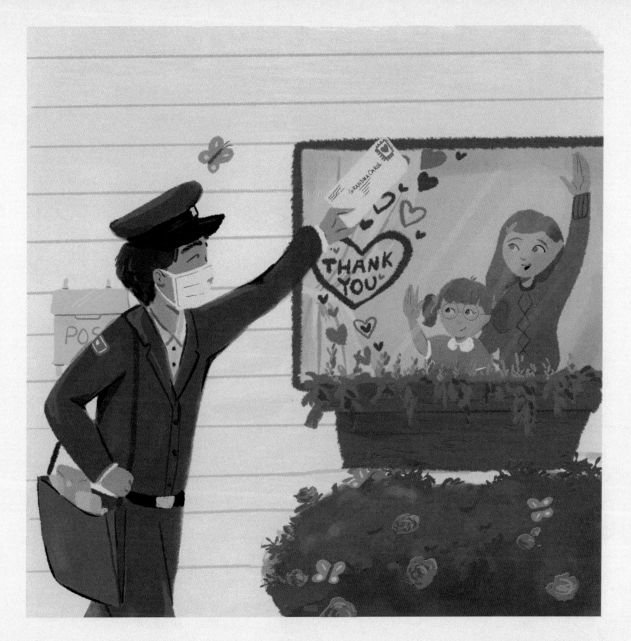

Heroes come in different, beautiful shapes and sizes, and not all of them wear capes. So, let's not forget to thank our heroes for being there for us. Who would you like to give thanks to?

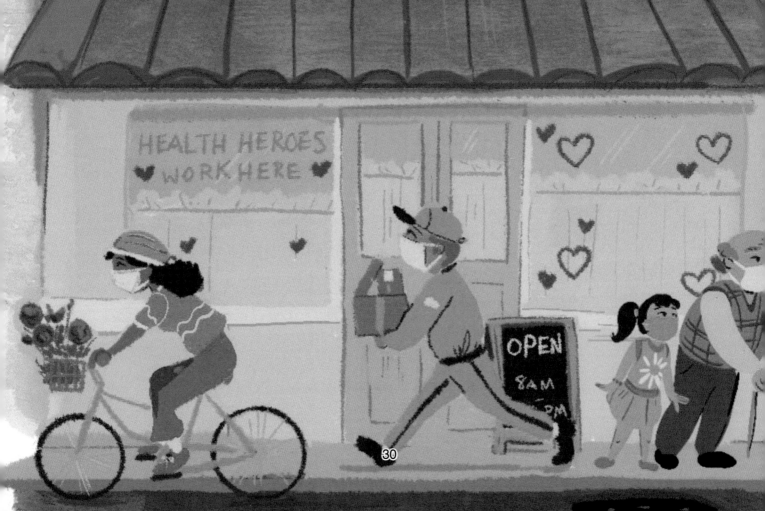

The world around us may not look the same as before, as it's going through some big changes that are affecting us all in different ways. Some of us can't see our close family and friends as much as we used to, go out to many places like before, and school is a bit different this year.

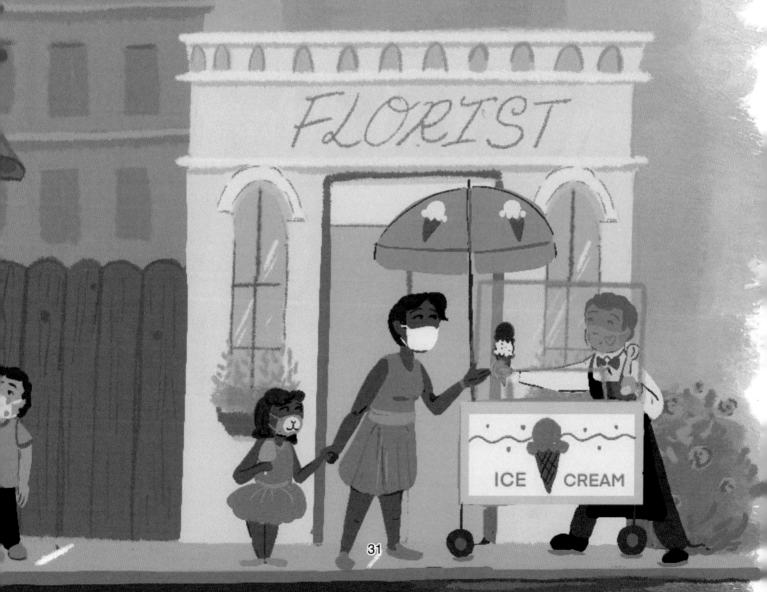

One thing is certain: the world around us will keep on going but so will we! Over time, you will see that the world presents challenges to you, but do not fear! Though it may be difficult to get through them on your own, don't forget to look around you. You will see that you are not alone, and there is a huge community of wonderful people ready to help you face any challenge. Because, in the end, a community grows stronger together.

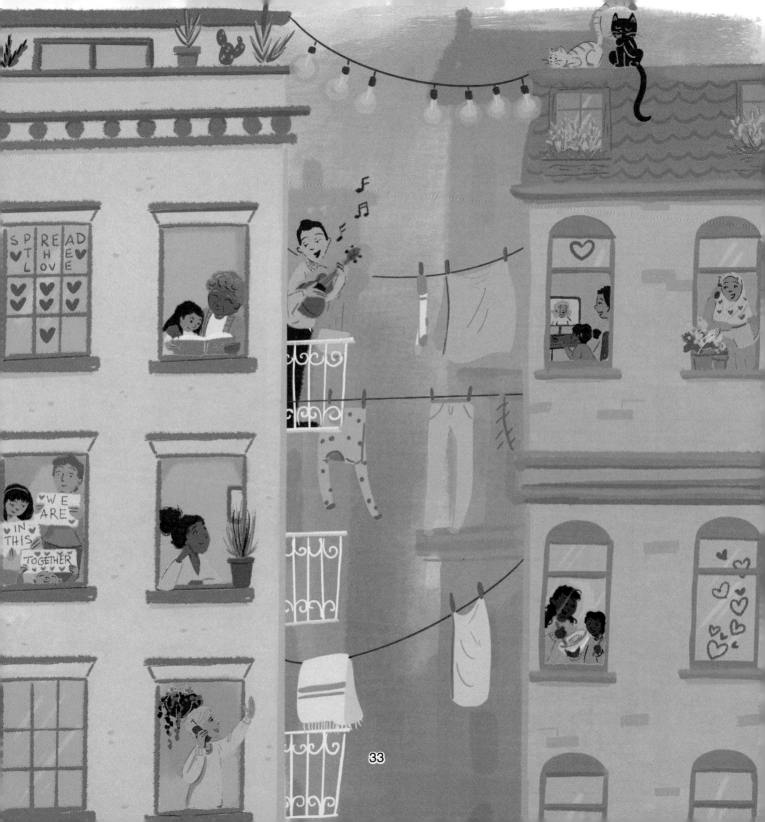

33

For the Kiddos...

Let's not forget the important essential steps for keeping bad germs away:

1. Cough and sneeze into your elbow or a tissue.
2. Wash your hands often. But for how long? 20 seconds silly!
3. Avoid touching your face.
4. When going to school or meeting up with a group of friends, don't forget to turn your bubble shield on (that means six feet apart)!
5. Wear a face mask or covering over your nose and mouth when in public or around people who don't live in your house.

For the Parents...

A few friendly tips on keeping your kids healthy:

1. Make handwashing a fun family activity.
2. Encourage your child to play outdoors. Physical activity and fresh air are not only great for physical health, but also for mental health.
3. Take breaks. Stretch, dance, and sing throughout the day to help your child stay healthy, happy, and focused.
4. Fingernails provide a sneaky hiding spot for icky germs. So clip your kids' nails more frequently.
5. Use hand lotion more often to avoid broken skin. Lotion will feel comfy and help prevent the spread of infections.

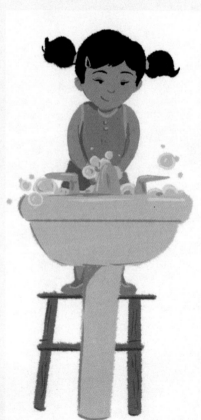

Friendly reminder: With everything going on in the world today, it may feel overwhelming. Try to make some time for yourself, and don't forget to let the good thoughts grow!

Real Facts about COVID-19 from the CDC website:

1. In the term COVID-19, 'CO' stands for 'corona,' 'VI' for 'virus,' and 'D' for disease. Formerly, this disease was referred to as the "2019 novel coronavirus" or "2019-nCoV."
2. Infections from the virus that causes COVID-19 have been reported in a small number of pets worldwide, including cats and dogs. The CDC recommends that even cats and dogs maintain a 6ft distance and avoid interaction such as those pictures in page 21.
3. People age 2 and older should wear masks that covers their noses and mouths in public settings and when around people who don't live in their household.
4. Choose a mask with two or more layers of washable, breathable fabric that fits snugly against the sides of your face.
5. If soap and water are not readily available, use a hand sanitizer that contains at least 60% alcohol content. Cover your entire hand surfaces with the sanitizer and rub your hands together until they feel dry.

The CDC is working with other federal partners on a comprehensive government response. This is an emerging, rapidly evolving situation and the CDC will continue to provide updated information as it becomes available. The CDC works 24/7 to protect people's health. More information about the CDC's response to COVID-19 is available online at **https://www.cdc.gov/.**

Excerpted information on COVID-19 excerpted from the Centers for Disease Control and Prevention website, provided for informational purposes only.

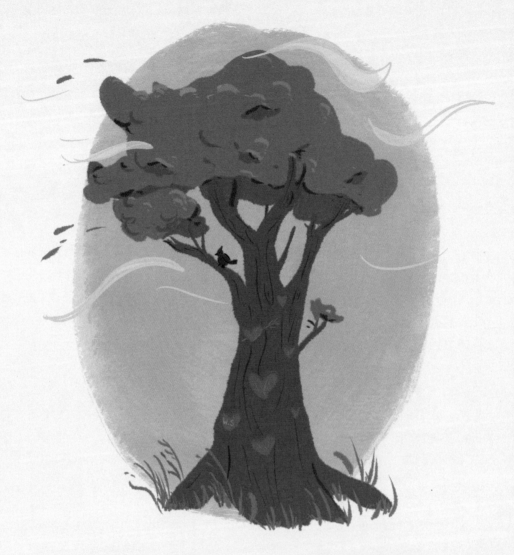

May this tree be dedicated to our loved ones
Who have been severely affected by the coronavirus
As we hope for strong recoveries. And to our loved ones who have succumbed to the
coronavirus, May they always be remembered through photos, cherished memories,
and warm hearts.

References

Center for Disease Control and Prevention. (2020, September 1). *About COVID-19.* https://www.cdc.gov/coronavirus/2019-ncov/cdcresponse/about-COVID-19.html

Center for Disease Control and Prevention. (2020, November 12). *Considerations for wearing masks: How to slow the spread of COVID-19.* https://www.cdc.gov/coronavirus/2019-ncov/prevent-getting-sick/cloth-face-cover-guidance.html

Center for Disease Control and Prevention. (2020, November 17). *COVID-19 and animals.* https://www.cdc.gov/coronavirus/2019-ncov/daily-life-coping/animals.html

Center for Disease Control and Prevention. (2020, November 4). *Hand sanitizer use out and about.* https://www.cdc.gov/handwashing/hand-sanitizer-use.html

Made in the USA
Middletown, DE
16 February 2021

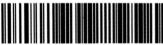